Ketogenic Diet

21 Days to Rapid Fat Loss, Laser Sharp Focus and a Better Life (Lose Up to A Pound A Day!)

Table of Contents

Introduction

Congratulations on downloading *Ketogenic Diet* and thank you for doing so.

The following chapters will discuss everything that you need to know about the Ketogenic Diet! This is a great diet for you to follow that is going to make it easier for you to gain control of your health.

With the Ketogenic Diet, you are going to be able to lose weight and gain energy better than with any other diet. While this may seem like another fad diet, this is one that has stuck around for a while, proving that it actually works.

Just like any diet, you are going to have to stick to it for a while in order to make sure that you can continue with it and are not going to be losing track; thus, causing you to fall off of the bandwagon and go back to your unhealthy way of living. Not only that, but you will want to pair this diet with exercise in order to get the weight off and keep it off!

There are plenty of books on this subject on the market, thanks again for choosing this one! Every effort was made to ensure it is full of as much useful information as possible. Please enjoy!

Chapter One: The Ketogenic Diet

It comes as no surprise that the Keto Diet is a diet! However, like all diets, there will be a reason behind why you choose to do a diet in the first place. You may be doing it because your food intake is high in protein, low in carbohydrates, or some other combination that is designed to assist you in losing weight, gaining muscle, or gaining energy.

When you are talking about the Ketogenic Diet, you will be talking about a low carbohydrate, high fat and adequate protein diet. The reason behind this is to force your body into burning the fat rather than the carbs that you are putting into your body. By doing this, you will see results in your waistline as it reduces in size. And who does not want that?

Before you can start this diet, your body is going to automatically begin taking carbohydrates in your food and turning it into glucose so that your body has the energy that you need to get through your day. However, in this diet you will be forcing your body to attack the fat cells and turn them into fatty acids, known as ketones, which will later be used as energy.

Most diets are going to require you to count calories and limit your calorie intake so that you can force your body to burn what it has already been given. Due to the calorie deficit, you will be causing your body to lose weight. This is the basic concept of weight loss. The Ketogenic Diet is going to work along the same lines. The fewer calories that you place in your body, the more your body will use what it is given. You are going to be training your body to realize that it has everything that it needs to produce energy already and that you are not going to have to constantly eat to have energy.

Any carbs that you put into your body will cause the blood glucose levels to become elevated. Whenever this happens, the insulin levels are going to rise as well. Since there is an increase of insulin in your body, it is going to be dispersed throughout your body which is going to cause you to feel hungry again. However, by limiting the number of carbs that you put into your body, this is going to keep your blood sugar levels steady. If you do not have the rapid spikes in insulin, you will be keeping yourself from feeling hungry shortly after you have already eaten. On top of that, you will be keeping your insulin levels low as your body is now going to be limiting how much fat it stores to promote an environment that is perfect for fat lipolysis.

Fat lipolysis is the process in which your body breaks down the fats in your body as well as the other lipids by hydrolysis in order to release the fatty acids.

Some people have reported that when they use the Ketogenic Diet, it is easy to restrict their calorie intake. There are a good majority of calories that are going to come from fats and proteins that you eat while you are on the Ketogenic Diet. This is going to make it to where you feel fuller longer, which is going to work better than limiting the number of calories you are consuming. When you remove simple carbs and refined sugar you will find that the number of calories that you eat in a day is going to be freed up for foods that will end up leaving you feeling full. You may even find that it is harder for you to reach your calorie goal by not having a false hope of being full because of foods that give you an empty feeling.

One of the biggest secrets behind the Ketogenic Diet is to balance your macronutrient ratios. There have been studies that show that users of the Ketogenic Diet will need to consume about sixty percent of their macronutrients from fat, another five percent from carbohydrates and the remaining thirty-five from protein.

When you start the Ketogenic Diet, it is highly recommended that you limit your carbohydrate intake to about twenty grams a day to push your body into a ketosis state. This is also going to help you learn how to be successful with a low carb diet. When your body is successfully placed into a ketosis state, you can up your intake of carbohydrates but it should remain under fifty grams per day.

During the first few weeks of your diet, you should keep track of everything that you eat and drink so that you know what is in the product and you can ensure that you are not putting too much of a single item into your body. With keeping track of all of the foods that you eat you are going to need to keep track of your calories as well. Since technology is so influential in our lives, there are a lot of apps that you can find that are going to work for you so that you can keep track of your food and calories.

As long as you stick to your diet, your body is going to get used to the restrictions that you place on it, therefore, it is going to be easier for you to understand the grams of carbs in the foods that you encounter and you will eventually adjust to where you live a low carbohydrate lifestyle. After you put your body into a state of ketosis, you will be able to raise your carb level to find your "sweet spot" and once you find that spot you will be keeping your body in a state of ketosis. Ensure that you are eating enough protein so that you are not doing harm to your body.

A major benefit that you will see with the Ketogenic Diet is that you are going to have more energy since you are keeping your insulin from spiking and your body is going to limit the fat that is stored which is going to result in you losing weight.

There are going to be recipes that you are going to be able to use in order to keep with your Ketogenic Diet. If you want to learn more about these recipes, look for the Ketogenic Cookbook!

You have to remember that with the Ketogenic Diet, you can really eat anything that you want. There are going to be some foods that you are going to want to stay away from which will be discussed in a later chapter, but, that is just so that you are not placing too much fat in your system. Other than that, you can eat anything and everything! How great is that?

Types of the Ketogenic Diet

Classic

Many dietitians are going to recommend the classic version based on the needs of the individual that will be following the diet. These recommendations will be based on food preferences, allergies, physical activities and culture. The classic Keto Diet will be good for an overwhelming majority of people.

Medium chain triglyceride (MCT)

MCT will be where you generate more ketos per unit of energy. When your diet is filled with MCT you will have less fat and more carbs and protein in your diet. An individual that wants to have more variety in their diet and portion sizes that are bigger than the normal ones that you will get with a diet.

Modified Atkins diet (MAD)

The MAD diet will be based on the Atkins diet for the most part, however, with it being modified you will notice that it is going to have a longer introduction phase where you will be intaking more fats and keeping a balanced diet. Just as with the Atkins diet, the diet will be put into place in order to control epileptic seizures.

Low glycemic index treatment (LGIT)

The lowered glycemic index diet is going to be when you are limiting other types. The concept behind this diet is to lower the intake of carbs while adding in extra fat. Should you have trouble controlling your blood glucose levels, this is going to be the Ketogenic Diet that you will follow.

Chapter Two: Benefits of the Keto Diet

1. The fat that is in your body will be used to fuel it so you can make it through the day. This is not going to happen if you are eating a lot of carbohydrates or if you are on a high carbohydrate diet. The more carbs that you put into your body, the more energy you will feel, but when your body reaches ketosis, then you have to force your body to become efficient by fueling itself to use the fat as energy.

2. Lowering how often you eat protein will make it to where you can take in the proper qualities of diet, instead of overdoing it or underdoing it like many people tend to do. At some point in time, you will place your body in ketosis and you will want less food which is going to lower the glucose in your system.

3. Since your body is not going to have all of the insulin in it, you will allow your hormones to stabilize as they are released in your body. There are some hormones that are going to be affected such as the growth hormones.

4. Ketones that enter your body during ketosis will make it to where you are not hungry as often. Which means you eat less.

5. When you cut carbohydrates, you are going to be losing weight. There are some studies that have shown that people who are on diets, where there are less carbs being eaten, lose weight faster. A reason for this is because a low carb diet tends to get rid of the extra water that is in your body. Since the insulin levels are lowered, your kidneys will be shredding the excess sodium leading to rapid weight loss in the first few weeks of the diet.

6. Not all body fat is going to be the same, and with a low carbohydrate intake you are going to realize that most of your fat is going to come from your abdominal cavity. The fat that you are going to lose more of is going to be the visceral fat that will hang out around your organs, and with a lot of fat there it is going to drive inflammation up. This is one of the biggest drivers for the metabolic dysfunctions that we see today. But a low-fat diet is going to get rid of a lot of the harmful fat that we put into our body. Not only that but it can help with other health issues that you may be experiencing.

7. The lower your triglyceride levels are, the lower your risk for heart disease will be.

8. Since low carbohydrate diets are high in fat; that is going to increase your HDL level, otherwise known as good cholesterol.

9. To lower blood sugar and insulin, you will reduce your carbohydrate consumption which may even be able to reverse type II diabetes.

10. There have been studies that show that when you reduce your carbs you will also be lowering your blood pressure which is one of the biggest risk factors for a lot of diseases that you see nowadays.

Chapter Three: What to Eat and What Not to Eat

It does not matter what type of diet that you are following, there are going to be things that you are going to want to avoid, so that you can achieve the goals that the diet is going to set for you. When you do the opposite of what the diet says then you will not be getting these results. Dieting can be frustrating, but with the Ketogenic Diet, you are not going to have this problem.

Wild animal and grass-fed animals

- Meat that has been grass fed is going to be better for everyone. Animals that are fed grass are going to be those that you find on a farm such as goat, lamb, cattle, and so on
- Any fish that has been caught in the wild or any seafood, but you are going to want to try and avoid any farmed fish
- Pork and poultry that is pastured
- Gelatin
- Butter
- Ghee
- Pastured eggs

Avoid

- Meat that is covered in breadcrumbs
- Sugary or starchy sauce meat
- Sausage
- Hot dogs
- The organ meats of grass fed animals such as the liver, kidneys and heart

Fats that are healthy for you

Saturated

- Lard
- Tallow
- Chicken fats
- Goose fats
- Duck fats
- Ghee
- Coconut oil
- Butter
- Clarified butter

Monounsaturated

- Olive oil
- Avocado oil
- Macadamia oil

Polyunsaturated

- Omega threes that are often found in seafood or fatty fish

Vegetables that do not have starch

Greens

- Lettuce
- Bok choy
- Swiss chard
- Chives
- Chard
- Spinach
- Radicchio
- Endive

Cruciferous vegetables

- Kale (the dark leaf one is the best for you)
- Radishes
- Kohlrabi

Other

- Cucumber
- Asparagus
- Celery stalks
- Summer squash
- Spaghetti squash
- Bamboo shoots
- Zucchini

Fruit

- Avocado

Condiments and beverages

- Water (of course, because it is one of the healthiest things that you can drink!)
- Tea (black tea and herbal tea are the best)
- Coffee (do not put creamer in it, though. If you cannot drink it black, then put cream or coconut milk in it for sweetness)
- Pork rinds are best for when you need to do breading
- Any spices or herbs
- Lime juice and zest
- Lemon juice and zest
- Mustard
- Pesto
- Mayonnaise
- Pickles
- Bone broth (you are going to want to make your own so that you can control what goes in it)
- Foods that are fermented (kimchi, sauerkraut (make your own) and kombucha)
- Whey proteins
- Egg whites

Eat sparingly

Vegetables, fruits, mushrooms

- Red cabbage
- White cabbage
- Green cabbage
- Broccoli
- Cauliflower
- Fennel
- Rutabaga
- Brussels sprouts
- Parsley root
- Leek
- Mushroom
- Onion
- Garlic
- Spring onion
- Winter squash
- Eggplant
- Peppers
- Tomatoes
- Bean sprouts
- Okra
- Kombu
- Nori
- Coconut
- Rhubarb

- Olives
- Sugar snap peas
- French artichokes
- Wax beans
- Water chestnuts
- Blackberries
- Strawberries
- Blueberries
- Cranberries
- Raspberries
- Mulberries

Grain fed animals and dairy

- Ghee
- Eggs
- Poultry
- Beef
- Try not to eat pork that is farmed because it is too high in omega 6s.
- Bacon (it has a lot of starch and preservatives)
- Full fat yogurt
- Sour cream
- Cheese
- Cottage cheese
- Try and avoid things that are low fat!

Nuts and seeds

- Brazil nuts (however, do not eat a lot of them because of the prominent level of selenium they contain)
- Hemp seeds
- Sunflower seeds
- Macadamia nuts
- Walnuts
- Almonds
- Pine nuts
- Flaxseed
- Sesame seeds
- Pumpkin seeds

Soy products

Try and stick with non-GMO soy products if you have to eat them. Fermented soy products are good too.

- Soy sauce
- Natto
- Tempeh
- Coconut aminos that are paleo friendly
- Green soy beans
- Black soybeans

Condiments

- Erythritol
- Swerve
- Stevia
- Arrowroot powder
- Xanthan gum
- Extra dark chocolate
- Carob powder
- Coco powder
- Ketchup
- Pureed tomatoes
- Passata tomatoes

Do not chew gum that is sugar free or suck on mints that are sugar free because where they do not have sugar, they have carbs.

Vegetables and fruits

- Carrots
- Sweet potato
- Beetroot
- Parsnip
- Celery root
- Honeydew melon
- Gallia melon
- Watermelon
- Cantaloupe

- Dragon fruit
- Apricot
- Peaches
- Cherries
- Pears
- Figs
- Plums
- Oranges
- Kiwi berries
- Kiwifruit
- Apples
- Nectarines
- Grapefruit

Alcohol

- Unsweet spirits
- Dry white wine
- Dry red wine

Avoid

These are the foods that you are going to want to avoid because they are meats that are factory farmed, food that is processed and rich in carbohydrates.

Grains

- Wholemeal
- Wheat
- Corn
- Rye
- Oats
- Millet
- Barley
- Bulgur
- Rice
- Sorghum
- Amaranth
- Rice
- Buckwheat
- Sprouted grains
- White potatoes
- Quinoa
- Pasta
- Pizza
- Cookies
- Bread
- Crackers
- Table sugar
- Ice cream
- Sweet pudding
- Agave syrup
- Soft drinks
- HFCS

Factory farmed fish and pork

- Fish that is high in mercury
- Fish inflamed with omega 6
- Fish with PCBs

Processed foods

- Food with carrageenan
- MSG
- BPAs
- Sulphites
- Artificial sweeteners
- Oils or fats that are refined
- Low carb products
- Zero carb products
- Low fat products
- Milk
- Sweet drinks
- Alcohol
- Tropical fruits
- Tropical fruit juices
- Tropical dried fruits
- Soy products (this is not just for the diet, but your health in general)
- Wheat gluten
- Carrageenan

In the event that you are not sure if you are allowed to have it, you will want to ask your doctor or just not eat it. Even if the list above says that it is alright for you to eat, it may not be. When in doubt, just leave it alone and eat something else!

Chapter Four: Keto Terms You Need to Know

As you learn about the Ketogenic Diet, there are terms that you will be hearing a lot and you should know what they mean. This is the section that will tell you about the terms and what they mean, so that you are not confused when you hear them later on.

- Keto (Keto Diet, Ketogenic Diet): a high fat, low carbohydrate diet that adds in moderate protein. It is named the Ketogenic Diet since you are forcing yourself to go into a state of ketosis.
- Paleo Diet: this is another diet that is going to be high in protein, low in carbs and moderate in fats. This diet is considered to be the diet that our ancestors followed and one of the easiest ways to describe it is if you cannot gather it or hunt it then you do not need to be placing it in your body.
- Total carbs and net carbs: net carbs will be your total carbs but will not include your fiber count. Whenever people are counting carbs, they will tell you that there is a right way and a wrong way, but there

is not. Count them in the way that you think is best for you.

- VLCKD (Very low carb Ketogenic Diet): just the name suggests you will be eating very little food with carbohydrates which means that you are going to eat around fifty grams of carbs a day.

- Zero carb diet: your Ketogenic Diet is not going to be anything like a zero-carbohydrate diet that you may have attempted before. Should you be following a zero-carb Keto Diet, then you are most likely eating about twenty grams a day. You have also most likely eliminated vegetables or are eating them in insignificant amounts. There is no proof that you will lose more weight when you do not eat any carbohydrates.

- Nutritional ketosis: nutritional ketosis will be when the ketones are between 0.5 and 0.3 mM. Your body will reach ketosis when your body stops forming glucose and is focusing on utilizing the fat in your system.

- Ketoacidosis: nutritional ketosis will be safe for your body but once you reach ketoacidosis you are going to experience health issues. Should you be an alcoholic or have type two diabetes, you will be at a higher risk of reaching ketoacidosis. Your body will end up having up to five times more ketones in your body when you reach this stage. If you have any health issues, you will need to talk to your doctor before starting the Ketogenic Diet.

- Exogenous ketones: synthetic ketones and the effects that they have on your health are still being studied. Normal exogenous ketones are going to enhance your performance if you are an athlete or they may help with some diseases. However, you will have to be careful with the products that have the ketones since they are typically marked incorrectly.

- Keto flu: during the first week or so while you are getting used to your diet, you are going to experience what people call the keto flu. You are not actually sick, but you will feel like you are. Your body is simply getting used to the fact that you are not eating as many carbohydrates as before. You can get over it by making sure that you keep your electrolytes up.

- Electrolytes: electrolytes are the sodium, potassium and magnesium levels that you will find in your body. They are overlooked when you are dieting; however, you need to make sure to manage your electrolytes so that you do not have effects such as the keto flu.

- Fat bomb: another thing that you may discover is hard when it comes to your diet is to manage the fat that you eat so that you eat healthy fats instead of the unhealthy kind; especially if you are new to dieting. Fat bombs will be the things that you eat that are high in fat and low in carbs and protein. These are small snacks that you may enjoy without worrying if you are breaking your diet or not.

Benefits of a fat bomb are:

- o Great party snacks
- o Help manage healthy fats
- o Snacks for before or after you work out
- o If you are trying to fast from fats

- Fat fast: it is going to take four weeks or more for your body to get used to your diet. Remember that before your body is used to the diet, you are going to be getting energy from glucose. Fat fasting will be for those who reached their place where they are no longer losing weight. During a fat fast, you will be getting most of your calories from healthy fat. If you do this, then you do not want to do it for more than five days or you can cause your body to go into starvation mode which is going to harm it.

- Beta-Hydroxybutyrate: BHB is a compound that is dissolved by the liver. The first of your ketones are going to be produced by fasting before you start your diet. You can use the blood ketone meter to measure the BHB that is in your system.

- Insulin resistance: insulin resistance is a condition where your cells are not going to handle the insulin in your body as they should. Whenever someone has IR they may end up having higher blood sugar or insulin levels. Should this be untreated, they can end up having diabetes or other autoimmune diabetes that are found in adults.

- Metabolic syndrome: at the point in time that you overcompensate your carbs you will end up with a metabolic syndrome known as hypertension, or various other health issues.

- Medium chain triglycerides: MCT are the saturated fats that our body is going to easily be able to use. They are mostly found in things like coconut oil and are going to be used differently by our body. The MCT are going to go straight to the liver and be converted into energy.

- Saturated fats: SFA are found in things like eggs, red meats, butter and ghee. They last longer on the shelf and are going to have high smoking point. Many of the oils that are used for cooking are going to be SFA. This is also where most of your fat intake should come from.

Chapter Five: Making the Keto Diet Easier

Starting a new diet is hard and with this chapter it is my goal to make it a little easier for you to be able to start your Ketogenic Diet. That way you are less likely to fall off the wagon later on, when it is tempting to; because it is hard for you to find something to eat or to remember that you have to manage your calorie intake.

Also, hopefully this will help you find it easier in making your meals Ketogenic friendly.

- Do you like butter? Well, you do not have to give it up! Just switch over to ghee. Ghee is similar to butter and can be used in recipes where butter normally would be.

- You are on a diet so you are going to need to make sure your body is getting everything that it needs. With the Ketogenic Diet, you will need plenty of omega threes.

- Try and stay away from alcohol. Not only is alcohol going to cause you to lose energy, but it is going to hinder your weight loss. Not to mention alcohol is not good for you.

- In a lot of recipes, you are going to find that you will need cream cheese. However, you will want to stay away from these recipes because there are a lot of carbs in cream cheese and when you eat a lot of cream cheese, you will be hindering your diet.

- Looking for something sweet to eat but you do not know what is healthy for your diet? Take heavy cream and some peanut butter. Mix them together and you will be creating a peanut butter mousse.

- Lemon water is going to keep your pH in balance and therefore you are going to want to drink it, especially while on the Keto Diet because your pH can become messed up while dieting.

- Low carb dark chocolate chips are great to have around if you crave something sweet.

- Traditional nonstick pans are not going to add flavor to your meat like a cast iron will; so, you may want to invest in a cast iron skillet.

- Do not add sugar to your cereal, instead, add some toasted coconut flakes.

- There are brands out there that have sugar free heavy whipping creams which are great when you are baking.

- If something is light or sugar free, then it is probably going to have more carbohydrates than the original ones.

- Don't bother changing your diet to low fats.

- While bacon is great, you do not want to eat too much of it!

- For extra energy, you will want to add some coconut oil.

- Water is great and is going to assist in your weight loss so you will want to drink plenty of it.

- Always preboil your eggs so you have a snack or even eggs so that you can make deviled eggs.

- Your carbs should be kept under twenty grams a day. You can up it if you need to but keep in mind that carbs are going to cause your body to store fat.

- Try and watch your protein intake. If you eat too much protein you will cause your insulin to spike.

- You do not want to have any cheat days if you want your diet to truly work. If you need one, you can take it, but you will have to work twice as hard to ensure your body stays in the ketosis state.

- Look to see how many carbs are in anything that you eat!

- Try and stay away from root vegetables. There are a lot of carbs in them.

- To get the salt that you need, you should drink chicken broth for the first two to three weeks so that you can keep your electrolytes up.

- Since your body is going to be changing, you should not exercise the first few weeks. Your body is already stressed and you do not want to stress it more. The only exception to this rule is if you are in a fitness program or an athlete.

- Take pictures of your progress and keep them where you are going to see them, so that you can see how far you have come.

This is going to make a difference and can keep you motivated when all hope feels like it has been lost or you are feeling discouraged.

- Make sure to keep yourself educated. There are different diets and nutrition facts that you will find about the diet to make your transition easier.

- Although you are limiting your body on certain foods, you do not need to do it for everything that you put in your body. Having a healthy serving of fat will not hurt you as long as you keep it in moderation. Think about eating things like seeds or avocados.

- Be patient! Switching around your way of life is going to take time and it is not going to happen right away. Therefore, you are not going to see results right away. However, if you stick to your diet longer you are going to see results. This is going to be a slow process.

- At the point in time you feel full, stop eating. There is no reason to overfill yourself at any meal. Eating more frequently is going to help keep your energy up and help you lose weight.

- You should also keep track of your body measurements along with your pictures. Sometimes, seeing the numbers makes it easier to keep going! You are going to see the numbers change before you begin to see it in your pictures.

- Plan your meals. This is going to help you know what you are putting into your body and you are not going to be tempted to go into the store and buy stuff that you should not be eating.

- Carbs are not evil, but you should make sure that you are moderating your intake of them. To do this, try and get rid of all the carby food that you have in your house. That way you can keep the cravings at bay. Out of sight, out of mind!

- Make just enough food for you to eat. Having leftovers is fine, but you do not want to make so much that you are going to be having the same meal for three weeks in a row.

- Should you have a cheat day or fall off the wagon, you do not have to beat yourself up. It is going to make it harder for your body to get back on track, but you can restart your diet and get back on the right path.

- Take responsibility for your own behavior. You should not use an excuse because you want to have something that you are not supposed to have. There are going to be plenty of reasons as to why you screw up, just own up to it and get yourself back to it as fast as possible.

- Another thing that you should keep a log of is when you fall of the wagon. This is going to assist you in making sure you can find your triggers and that way you can stay away from them.

- Try to restart your diet when you slip. Eat a salad or do not eat at all. That way you can get your body back into the swing of being on the diet.

- Find someone who can help you and be supportive in making sure that you stick to your diet. When you have someone there, you can go to them when you want something that is not going to be good for your diet. Not only will you be helping yourself, but you will be helping them as well.

- Fasting is not going to be bad when on the Keto Diet. You should take intermittent periods where you fast but keep yourself hydrated. You will want to take a twelve to sixteen-hour time period where you are cleansing and then eight to twelve hours of building. The more that you follow this pattern, the easier it is going to be to ensure your body is in ketosis.

- If you are going to exercise, then you need to have a routine schedule of what you are going to do, when it is going to be done and how long you will be doing it. You are not going to want to stress your body any more than you have to and exercise was created to stress the body. You should try and keep the exercise to do after you have gotten used to the Ketogenic Diet.

- Keep your stress down as much as you can. Whenever you stress, your body is going to release hormones that are going to elevate your blood sugar and this is going to be similar to when your insulin is released because of hormones.

- Change how you sleep. You will need to get plenty of sleep in order to lose weight and increase your energy levels. Not only that, but you are going to be lowering your stress levels. One of the best ways to sleep is to place the temperature in your room between 60 – 65 degrees. Cool air encourages your body to relax so that you stay asleep longer. You may also want to sleep with a mask on to block out the light. Should you find that you are having trouble sleeping, melatonin will help, or even ear plugs if you are going to be around loud noises during your hours of sleep.

Chapter Six: The Efficiency of the Ketogenic Diet

With the Ketogenic Diet, studies have shown that seizures in patients have been reduced by about fifty percent of those who try the diet, and reduces them by ninety percent in a third of patients. Around three quarters of children who follow the Ketogenic Diet respond within two weeks despite the fact that experts have recommended a trial of around three months before they see if it has been effective or not. Children who suffer from refractory epilepsy are probably going to benefit more from a Ketogenic Diet instead of attempting to place them on another anticonvulsant drug. There has even been evidence that teenagers and adults may benefit from the diet as well.

Trial design

Some of the earlier studies that have been completed have shown a high success rate. In a study done in 1925, around sixty percent of patients eventually became seizure free while another thirty-five patients had their seizure frequency reduced by fifty percent. In these studies, generally, a cohort of patients were examined because they had recently been treated by physicians (this is known as a retrospective study). The patients were selected by the fact that they were able to maintain the proper dietary restrictions. But, these studies are difficult to compare to more modern trials. One of the reasons would be because the older trials suffer from selection bias since they excluded patients who could not start or could not maintain the diet, and so patients were selected who would give better results. To try and control any bias in a modern-day study, a prospective cohort (patients are selected before the study begins) so that the results that are present for all patients will be given even if the patient could not start or complete the treatment. This is also known as intent to treat analysis.

Another difference that you are going to see between the older studies and the innovative studies, is that there is a different type of patient that is being treated with the Ketogenic Diet. When the studies first started, the diet was not a treatment of last resort. But, looking at modern studies, children have already used an untold number of drugs to try and treat their seizures and they end up being diagnosed with a difficulty to treat epilepsy. Both early and modern studies are going to differ because the treatment protocol has changed. With older protocols, a diet was started with a prolonged fast so that the patient could lose five to ten percent of their body weight and then they would be heavily restricted on the calories they took in. There were concerns about child health and growth that later led to a relaxation of the diet's restrictions. Fluid restrictions were also a feature of the diet, but this ended up causing patients to be constipated or have kidney stones and it is no longer considered beneficial to the study.

Outcomes

A study that was started with the intent to treat prospective was first published in 1998 by a team of doctors that were working at the Johns Hopkins Hospital, this study was followed up and a report published later in 2001. Just like most studies that have been done on the Ketogenic Diet, there is not going to be a control group. This study in particular, took a hundred and fifty children and examined them for three months. After those three months, eighty three percent were still following the diet as they were supposed to, twenty-six of them were experiencing a reduction in seizures, thirty one percent had a major education of seizures, and three percent showed that they were seizure free. After a year the numbers lowered, but the number of those that were no longer experiencing seizures had increased. The patients that were no longer following the diet decided to do so because it showed to be ineffective due to illness. Even as the study continued, some of the numbers were lowered while those who were benefiting from the study increased. At this time in the study, children dropped out of it because they were seeing a good reduction in the frequency of their seizures or because they were now seizure free. After four years, all one hundred and fifty children either saw less seizures occurring or they were not seeing them at all. The children who stayed on the diet all through the four years would not necessarily be seizure free, but they did experience superior results with the diet!

There is always the possibility that you can combine results from multiple small studies that have given you outcomes that are stronger together than they are when they are alone. This is a statistical method known as meta-analysis. At least one of four analysis that were conducted back in 2006 took nineteen studies consisting of over a thousand patients just to conclude that at least fifty percent of the patients reached a reduction of fifty percent in their seizure frequency. While, at the same time, a third of those patients showed a ninety percent reduction.

A review that was done in 2012 discovered and then analyzed for randomly controlled trials that were using the Ketogenic Diet in children that experienced epilepsy. These trials were done when drugs were no longer working or had failed to control their seizures. In one of the trials it compared a group that was assigned the diet and another group that was not. In other trials, they compared the diets or other ways that a diet could be introduced in order to make it more tolerable by the patient. Around forty percent of the kids had fewer seizures when they were following a strict diet. But, only ten percent were still on the diet a few years later. Some of the adverse effects such as loss of energy or hunger were common as was constipation, which could be found in around thirty percent of the patients in the study.

Chapter Seven: Adverse Effects of the Keto Diet

It is vital that you are aware of the adverse effects of the Ketogenic Diet because if you begin to experience these symptoms, you can go to your doctor to find a way to modify your diet or something else that is going to be the solution to the problem that you may be experiencing. This diet is not holistic, benign, nor is it a natural treatment for any serious medical condition, there may be complications when the diet is used as treatment as we have discussed in the previous chapter.

The Ketogenic Diet is likely to assist in causing seizures to be less frequent and less severe than if a patient was on anticonvulsant medication or had to undergo surgery. Some of the more easily treatable complications are going to be things such as constipation, hypoglycemia, or low-grade acidosis. However, these complications are generally going to be some of the less severe affects that can be seen in patients using the Ketogenic Diet for seizures.

In the event that a fast happens before the diet is actually started, the patient may experience a rapid rise in their lipid levels which has been known to affect up to sixty percent of those who have participated in a ketogenic study. Along with that, their cholesterol levels may increase. These affects can be treated with a change in the fat content of the diet. But, if the affect continues, the ketogenic ratio will be lowered. One other change could be to add in supplements for the diet due to the fact that there is a dietary deficiency.

Sadly, the long-term effects of using the diet over a prolonged period of time can cause slow or stunted growth in children, kidney stones, and bone fractures. This diet may reduce the levels of insulin such as the growth factor number one, and this insulin is vital to childhood growth. Much like the anticonvulsant medications that seizure patients take, the Ketogenic Diet is going to affect one's bone health. There are other factors that will be involved such as acidosis.

Around one in twenty patients (particularly children) who are on the Ketogenic Diet have developed kidney stones. One of the classes of anticonvulsant medications known as carbonic anhydrase inhibitors has been known to increase kidney stones; however, the combination of the drug and the diet have not shown to elevate the risk. While kidney stones are treatable and do not show any need to discontinue the diet, the Johns Hopkins hospital has begun to give out potassium citrate supplements to anyone who is following the Ketogenic Diet under their instruction. This simple supplement has shown to decrease the incidence of kidney stones almost sevenfold. But, this treatment has not officially been studied in a controlled trial. While following the Ketogenic Diet, there are at least four reasons as to why you may be experiencing kidney stones.

- There is an excess of calcium in the patient's urine because of an increased bone demineralization; thanks to acidosis. Since bones are made mostly of calcium phosphate, the phosphate will react to the acid and cause the calcium to be excreted by the kidneys.
- Hypocitraturia which is when there is a low concentrate of citrate in the body which is usually used to dissolve free calcium.
- Whenever the urine has a low pH, the uric acid stops dissolving, which can lead to crystals which in turn turns into calcium stones otherwise known as kidney stones.
- There are plenty of institutions that restrict the intake of water to patients on diets by eighty percent, however, because of kidney stones. This practice is no longer encouraged and is rarely used.

Some teenagers and adults have even reported that they experienced dyslipidemia while a few women have experienced dysmenorrhea.

Chapter Eight: Implementing the Keto Diet from a Medical Point of View for Seizures

The Ketogenic Diet is a nutritional therapy that is used by medical professionals. The diet is going to involve participants of various disciplines. There are team members that are going to include a pediatric dietitian, neurologist, a registered nurse, and maybe even a social worker and pharmacist. Each person involved in the study is going to be aware of how the diet is going to work in children as well as how to make it work for the child participant in an effort to lower if not get rid of the seizures that the child experiences.

When the diet is implemented, it can present some difficulties to not just the patient, but the caregiver as well because of how much time and commitment is involved in planning each meal. Any unplanned eating would end up breaking the nutritional balance that is required; therefore, some people actually have the discipline to maintain the challenges that the diet is going to bring up. There are some people who end up terminating the diet or modifying it since the difficulties are too great.

Initiation

The protocol that is followed at Johns Hopkins hospital has drastically changed and has begun the initiation of the Ketogenic Diet to be widely adopted. This adaptation involves a consultation with the patient and their parents or caregiver as well as a stay at the hospital. Due to the complications that could arise with the Ketogenic Diet being used, a lot of hospitals are going to require that the patient stay and start their diet under the close supervision of a medical professional. That way if issues are going to occur, they can catch it before it is too late.

During the first consultation, patients are going to be screened to see if there are any conditions that may cause the diet to be a bad idea. There is going to be a dietary history obtained as well as the parameters that are going to arise for the diet that has been selected. This is where the diet will be modified to fit the patients' needs and ensure that it is going to work the way that it is supposed to.

Before the patient is admitted to the hospital there are going to be some drop-in carbohydrates in the diet so that the patient can begin to fast after they eat their evening meal. Once admitted, they are only going to get caffeine and calorie free fluids until their evening meal. Slowly, they are going to be introduced to the Ketogenic Diet to allow their body to adapt to the changes. On the day that they are discharged, they are going to be on solid foods and hopefully carbohydrate free medications.

As the patient is in the hospital, their glucose levels will be checked multiple times a day so that they can be checked for symptomatic ketosis. While a lack of energy and lethargy are common, they tend to vanish inside of two weeks. The caregiver will attend classes to make sure that they know how to properly administer the diet and medications that are needed for the diet. This is also meant to help answer any questions the caregiver may have about ensuring that their child gets enough of what the diet requires to ensure that they are getting the proper results. There will be some questions that are going to require private consultations with the attending physician especially if there are special conditions due to the patient's condition and medical needs.

It's common for protocol to change to fit the patients' needs as they continue to follow the diet as an outpatient. Sometimes there may be no need for a fast since fasting increases the risk of hypoglycemia and acidosis. Other times the portion sizes of the meals will vary.

There are some people who have shown seizure reduction within the first five days of the diet being implemented. More have shown a reduction in the first two weeks, while about ninety percent show a reduction in the first twenty-three days. Should the diet not start with a fast, then the time is going to be longer for patients to show an improvement in their seizures.

Maintenance

Once the diet has started, the child who is participating in the diet will visit a doctor regularly as well as a dietitian and a neurologist to go through various tests to make sure that the diet is not harming them. These checks are going to happen even three months during the first year and then will spread out more as the diet is continued. Visits may be more frequent should there be special medical conditions or because of the age of the child. There is going to be an adjustment period like there will be for anything new introduced into someone's life. But, with the Ketogenic Diet, it will be to make sure ketosis has been reached.

There may be an increase of seizures when the subject is ill or should their ketone levels fluctuate. This diet can be modified should the frequency of seizures remain high or if the subject is losing too much weight.

Discontinuation

Around twenty percent of those on the Ketogenic Diet have made it to a point where they are free from seizures and can either reduce the number of drugs that they are taking or can get rid of them altogether. Around two years of strictly following the diet can cause the patient to be seizure free and the diet may be slowly discontinued after two to three months of there being no seizures.

Getting off the diet will require that the ketogenic ration is lowered until the urinary ketosis can no longer be detected. After that, the calorie restrictions can be lifted. The timing is going to mimic how patients are taken off their anticonvulsant meds when they become seizure free. However, should a patient be taken off the Ketogenic Diet completely if at all will be up to the caregiver and the medical team that is attending to that patient.

Chapter Nine: The Keto Diet and Diabetes

As you follow the Ketogenic Diet, it can potentially lower your blood glucose levels. While you manage your carbohydrate intake, it is recommended that if you suffer from type two diabetes since carbohydrates are turned into sugar and when ingested in large quantiles, it can cause your blood sugar to spike. So, if you suffer from high blood glucose, when you eat too many carbs you are going to be placing yourself in danger. Looking at the other side of things, when you focus on fat, you will experience the reduction in blood sugar that you will be looking for.

Potential dangers

While you are changing your primary source of energy, you are going to be increasing the ketones in your blood. Dietary ketosis will be different from ketoacidosis which as you know is dangerous from previous chapters. Whenever you place too many ketones in your body you will be placing yourself at risk for diabetic ketoacidosis. Diabetic ketoacidosis is prevalent when dealing with type one diabetes whenever blood glucose happens to be too high, which can come from a lack of insulin. Diabetic ketoacidosis is rare, but it is possible it can happen when you are dealing with type two diabetes should the ketones be too high. If you are sick while you are following a low carbohydrate diet, you may increase your risk for diabetic ketoacidosis.

While you are on the Ketogenic Diet, you need to make sure that you are testing your blood sugar to ensure that they are staying inside of their range. You may also want to test to make sure you are not placing yourself at risk for diabetic ketoacidosis. It is recommended by the American Diabetes Association that you test your ketones in the event that your blood sugar is two hundred and forty mg/dL. You will be able to test your ketones at home with urine strips to make sure that it has not gotten too high.

If at any point in time you see that you are experiencing symptoms of diabetic ketoacidosis, then you need to take yourself to the emergency room because you will be experiencing a medical emergency. The symptoms of diabetic ketoacidosis are:

- consistently high blood sugar
- dry mouth
- frequent urination

- nausea
- breath that has a fruit-like odor
- breathing difficulties

Monitoring your diabetes

As much as we have discussed the Ketogenic Diet in this book, it should seem pretty straight forward. But, unlike some low-calorie diets, a high fat diet will require you to monitor it carefully. There may even be some circumstances where you will start the diet in the hospital under medical supervision so that your blood glucose and ketone levels can be monitored to make sure that you are keeping the appropriate levels for them and that you are not experiencing adverse effects. After your body has adjusted to the diet, you will need to continue to visit your doctor to see if there are modifications that need to be made to your diet or medication.

It does not matter if your symptoms improve, it is important that you continue to test your blood glucose regularly. When you suffer from type two diabetes, monitoring will be different in how frequently you test. It is going to be up to your doctor so that the best schedule can be determined for testing.

Research on the Ketogenic Diet and diabetes

Back in 2008, researchers took twenty-four weeks to study how a low carbohydrate diet effected people who were obese and those who suffer from type two diabetes. When the study came to an end, they saw that those who followed the diet saw greater improvements when it came to their control over their glycemic levels as well as the possibility of reducing their medication compared to someone who decided to follow a low glycemic diet. Later on, in 2017, the Ketogenic Diet was proven to outperform normal low-fat diabetes diets that span over thirty-two weeks when it came to weight loss and A1c levels.

Outlook

Following the Ketogenic Diet may offer some hope to someone who suffers from type two diabetes as they have difficulties controlling their symptoms. One benefit is that they are going to experience few diabetic symptoms even if they are still depending on medications, although they may be able to lower their medications and eventually get off them altogether. However, it may be likely that you may not experience success with this diet. The restrictions may be too difficult for some people. But, keep in mind that if you yo-yo between diets that you are going to be placing yourself in danger of throwing your blood sugar levels off. So, if you start the Ketogenic Diet, you need to stick to it to ensure that you are getting the full benefits of the diet.

Chapter Ten: Steps to Starting a Ketogenic Diet

All throughout this book you have seen how a Ketogenic Diet is helpful to assist in various medical issues, particularly seizures. However, how do you start a Ketogenic Diet if you are not requiring that a medical professional supervise you?

First of all, you are still going to want a doctor to know that you are following the diet in the first place so that you can have someone who can watch for signs of ketoacidosis. Not only that, but it could bring up medical issues that you are unaware of and that have to be treated.

Step one: consult your doctor.

While a Ketogenic Diet is based on medical and nutritional facts, there is not one opinion in the medical community that the diet is effective for weight loss. Consult your medical doctor to see if the diet is right for you.

There are going to be some sources that say that the Ketogenic Diet is good to treat medical illnesses instead of weight loss.

Should you happen to be pregnant or diabetic, your doctor will closely monitor your diet and medications to ensure that everything is working out the way that it is supposed to.

Someone who is a type one diabetic will need to also seek medical treatment before beginning this diet.

Step two: recognize the risks for the diet.

Since the Ketogenic Diet is gong to be placing your body into ketosis, you are going to be putting yourself at risk, especially if you suffer from heart or kidney problems. If you suffer from any heart diseases or kidney diseases you should avoid the Keto Diet all together because of the strain that it will be placing on your kidneys.

Step three: start with a general low carb diet.

The Atkins diet is a diet that is based heavily on fats and proteins while remaining low on carbs and is going to be just the diet that is going to slowly show your body how to burn ketones for the energy that it needs. You do not have to do this, though, it is just to make the transition period easier on you and your body.

Step four: calculate your macronutrients.

These are the nutrients that your body will require in large quantites in order to form calories. When you calculate your intake of macronutrients you are going to be able to see your level of fat consumption. By knowing this information you will be able to decide how to reduce your carbohydrate and protein consumption while increasing fat.

Step five: eat about twenty to thirty grams of carbs a day.

By using a macronutrient calculator you will be able to eat more than thirty grams of carbs a day, however, you need to decrease your carbohydrate intake so that you can burn ketones and give yourself more energy.

About ten percent of your daily calories will come from carbs.

When you focus on carbs, look towards non-starchy vegetables and salad greens while avoiding pasta and bread.

Step six: eat up to eight ounces of protein a day.

Protein is a vital part of your diet and if you do not have any protein you are not going to have any energy which will cause you to feel hungry or develop cravings. But, if you have too much protein you will not be able to experience the weight loss effects that comes from the Ketogenic Diet.

You need to try and consume about thirty percent of your daily calories in protein. How much protien you eat is going to depend on how much you need on an individual basis which will be tied to your lifestyle.

Step seven: eat fat with every meal.

Go back to our chapter on foods that you can eat and foods that you should stay away from. Choose fats off of the list so that you can enjoy one with each meal that you eat. Fats are going to encourage the burning of fatty ketones for fuel.

Step eight: do not stress about calories.

You are not going to have to actively keep track of your calories, but it is recommended. This recommendation comes from the atempt of lowering your food cravings that you are going to experience.

You should be intaking:

1050 calories of fat

150 calories of carbs

300 calories of protein

Step nine: stay hydrated.

Your kidneys are going to get rid of extra water in your body which means that you are going to have to replace it. This is so that you can avoid dehydration. If you experience muscle cramps or headaches you may be experiencing dehydration.

Deyhydration may also mean you need to increase your salt and magnesium intake.

Step ten: measure your ketones.

A ketone meter is going to take some blood and see where your blood sugar is which will tell you if you are in ketosis or not. There are certain ketones that can measure urine instead of blood, but testing blood is going to be more accurate. You can find a ketone meter in a drug store.

Step eleven: look for signs of the keto flu.

You may experience high energy, mental clarity, strong smelling breath or urine, nausea, or no appitite, and these are all going to be signs of the keto flu. If you are experiencing any of these symptons you should go to your doctor and see if you need to modify your diet. But that will only occur if you have not seen these symptoms vanish once you have become keto adapted.

Chapter Eleven: The Keto Diet vs The Paleo Diet

When you look at the Paleo Diet it is going to represent a long term diet plan, however, the Ketogenic Diet is going to get rid of most of the calories you eat from fat in a shorter period of time.

Whenever you break it down from the perspective of food, both diets are going to require that you avoid processed foods and grains, but the Paleo Diet is going to go a step further and get rid of dairy. The Keto Diet is also going to advise that you stay away from fruits, tubers, and sweet vegetables unlike the Paleo Diet. Both diets are going to include meat, healthy fat, poultry, fish, nuts and seeds, along with non starchy vegetables.

How else do the diets differ? Well, the Ketogenic Diet is going to focus on the manipulation of protein, carbs, and fats while the Paleo Diet will lean more towards healthy choices and a larger balance of macronutrients.

How do the proteins line up?

For both diets, the proteins are going to be similar, but the Paleo Diet will be stricter because they want you to lean more on plant based proteins while avoiding lentils, beans, peanuts, and other legumes.

Fat

The Keto Diet is going to encourage a high intake of fat and make it to where you can eat vegetable oils and dairy products. But, the dairy and fat products should not be hydrogenated such as margarine. With all the information out there today, you can see the harmful effects that some vegetable oils are going to have.

The Paleo Diet will tell you to avoid these all together and once again is going to push you towards plant based fats. This diet also is an advocate for grass fed animal products.

Low carb

Since both diets are going to focus on eating enough protein and fat, they are going to require less carbohydrates. The Paleo Diet allows for carbs from carrots, and other root vegetables while these vegetables need to be avoided while follwoing the Ketogenic Diet.

Fruit

The Keto Diet is going to highly discourage you from having any fruit because of the sugar, glucose, and fructose content. Both glucose and fructose are going to contribute to weight gain and cause you to become insulin resistant. The biggest exception that you are going to find is the berries that contain antioxidants so that you can balance out the sugar content.

The Paleo Diet on the other hand is going ot support you eating almost any type of fruit that you can get your hands on.

Other facts

1.   The ultimate goal
Keto: weight loss
Paleo: better health

2.   Carb level
Keto: low
Paleo: varies

3. Dairy?
Keto: yes!
Paleo: no, because of inflammation and other health issues

4. Tofu?

Keto: yes, because it is low carb

Paleo: no, because it is soy and is believed to cause inflammation.

5. Sweet potatoes?

Keto: no, since they are high in carbs

Paleo: yes, since they are toxin free and full of nutrients

6. Wheat based soy sauce?

Keto: depending on the Keto Diet you are following it is on the list of things that you can use because it does not have a lot of carbs

Paleo: no, since it is going to irritate the gut being that it is soy

7. Fruit?

Keto: no, it is full of sugar

Paleo: yes!

Which one is better?

Looking at the break down of each diet, it is hard to tell which one is going to be better without first examining your own health. There are benefits from each diet and there are also limitations that have to be put into place. Both diets can be modifed for an individual and can have add ons that are going to burn fat, prevent or treat disease, and lower blood sugar.

One compromise is to follow the hunter gather lifestyle which is going to be a little harder in todays world, but can be done; while the other is going to allow you to look at everything you eat and basically allow you to eat anything that you want as long as you follow a very basic outline of food.

Either way, if you want to know which one is best for you, you need to go to your doctor and have a discussion with them to find the one that is the perfect fit for you personally.

Chapter Twelve: Basic Recipes

For this chapter you will see a few recipes that are going to show you what you are going to be looking for when you are dealing with ketogenic diet. However, for more in depth recipes you are going to want to download the Keto Cookbook which will take you into recipes that you can make for any occassion at all times of the day!

Flaxseed Crackers and Keto spinach and artichoke dip

What you need:

- Flax seeds (1 cup)
- Red pepper flakes (1/2 teaspoon, optional)
- Water (1 cup)
- Onion powder (1/2 teaspoon, optional)
- Rosemary (1 teaspoon, optional)
- Garlic powder (1/2 teaspoon, optional)

What to do:

1. Dump flax seeds into a bowl. Put in the fridge for up to eighteen hours.
2. Take the flax seeds and place them on a sheet of parchment paper. Roll as thin as you can get them.
3. Your oven needs to be set to 275F and the seeds cooked for an hour on the paper they are sitting on.

Keto spinach and artichoke dip

What you need:

- Salt and pepper (to taste)
- Cream cheese (8 ounces)
- Mozzarella cheese (8 ounces)
- May (1/4 cup)
- Spinach (255 grams)
- Parmesan (4 ounces, shredded)
- Artichoke hearts (14 ounces)
- Garlic (1 tablespoon, minced)
- Basil (1 teaspoon, crushed)

What to do:

1. Set your cream cheese in a microwave-safe bowl and melt it down.
2. Now mix the mayo.
3. Add in the parmesan and seasonings.
4. Take the artichoke hearts and cut them down.
5. Take a pan that is roughly 8x8 and grease it before you dump your dip into the bottom.
6. Sprinkle the mozzarella cheese over the top.
7. Cook for around thirty minutes at 350 F.

Cheesy beef balls

What you need:

- Cheddar (cubed, 12, optional)
- Ground beef (1.5 cups)
- Cheddar cheese (shredded, 0.75 cups)

What to do:

1. Combine the beef and the cheese.
2. Roll into twelve balls of equal size.
3. If you are placing the cubed cheese in the middle, make sure that you do this before you roll them into balls.
4. Deep fry them at 375 F.

Beef Brussels sprouts

What you need:

- Pepper (to taste)
- Brussels sprouts (3 cups)
- Ground beef (2 cups)
- Fish sauce (2 ounces)
- Oil or bacon grease (2 ounces)

What to do:

1. Take the stems out of the Brussels sprouts and cut into quarters.
2. Mix the sprouts into the oil.
3. Cook the ground beef until there is no pink left.
4. Add this into the mixture along with your seasoning.
5. Place in a pan that has been greased.
6. For forty minutes, cook at 450 F.
7. Stir them every ten minutes.
8. Boil them for a few minutes before enjoying.

Mini pepper nachos

What you need:

- Tomato (chopped, .5 cups)
- Chili powder (1 tablespoon)
- Cheddar cheese (shredded (1.5 cups)
- Cumin (ground, 1 teaspoon)
- Mini peppers (seeded, halved, 16 ounces)
- Garlic powder (1 teaspoon)
- Ground beef (16 ounces)
- Paprika (1 teaspoon)
- Red pepper flakes (.25 teaspoon)
- Salt (kosher, .5 teaspoon)
- Oregano (.5 teaspoon)
- Pepper (.5 teaspoon)

What to do:

1. Mix seasonings together in a bowl.
2. On medium heat, brown the meat to be sure all the clumps are broken up.
3. Mix in the spices and continue to sauté until the seasoning has gone through all of the meat.
4. Heat the oven to 400 F.
5. Place the peppers in a single line. They can touch.
6. Coat with beef mix.
7. Sprinkle with cheese.
8. Bake for around ten minutes or until cheese has melted.
9. Pull out of the oven and top with the toppings.

Beef stroganoff

What you need:

- Spaghetti squash (1.5 cups)
- Beef (cubed, 56 ounces)
- Sour cream (1 cup)
- Olive oil (2 tablespoons but you may need more)
- Red wine (0.25 cups)
- Flour (0.75 cups)
- Beef stock (1.25 cups)
- Salt (kosher, 1 teaspoon)
- Garlic (minced, 3 cloves)
- Pepper (.5 teaspoon)
- Onion (sliced, 1)
- Onion powder (.5 teaspoon)
- Paprika (0.125 teaspoon)
- Thyme (dried, .5 teaspoon)
- Rosemary (dried, .5 teaspoon)

What to do:

1. Mix together the seasonings in a zip lock bag.
2. Add in beef and shake until thoroughly coated.
3. Put in pressure cooker and allow to brown.
4. Add in oil.
5. When the beef has browned, remove it.

6. Place onions and more oil in, allowing the onions to cook for about five minutes

7. Next, add in the garlic.

8. Replace the meat and any juices that you may have collected on your plate.

9. Add beef stock and wine to the mixture.

10. Cover and cook for twenty minutes.

11. Place the sour cream in a bowl.

12. Move some of the juice from the pressure cooker to the bowl with the sour cream and stir until mixed and the sour cream has become warm.

13. Now stir this into the meat mixture.

14. Serve over vegetable noodles that you made earlier.

Conclusion

Thank you for making it through to the end of *Ketogenic Diet*, let's hope it was informative and able to provide you with all of the tools you need to achieve your goals whatever they may be.

The next step is to start your diet! You are going to find that it is hard for you to start it at first, especially if you are not used to dieting. But, you are going to be able to do it as long as you put your mind to it! Try to do everything you can to stay motivated and stick to the diet. You will be glad you did.

Finally, if you found this book useful in any way, a review on Amazon is always appreciated!

Thank you and good luck!